AETCOM

Attitude, EThics and COMmunication

MANUAL

Learning Modules for MBBS Professional Year II
Competencies for the
Indian Medical Graduate

As Recommended by National Medical Commission

AETCOM

Attitude, EThics and COMmunication

MANUAL

Learning Modules for MBBS Professional Year II
Competencies for the
Indian Medical Graduate

As Recommended by National Medical Commission

Nitin Ashok John
MBBS MD FRSB (London, UK), FASSOPI (India), FAcad Med Edu (Cardiff, UK), FRSPH (London, UK 2021),
PGDMLE (Medical Law and Ethics, NLSIU Bengaluru), DIH, PGDHA (Hospital Administration)
MA (Public Administration), European Life Style Medicine Organization Certified Graduate

Professor and Head
Department of Physiology
All India Institute of Medical Sciences
Bibinagar, Hyderabad

CBSPD

CBS Publishers & Distributors Pvt Ltd

New Delhi • Bengaluru • Chennai • Kochi • Kolkata • Lucknow • Mumbai
Gujarat • Hyderabad • Jharkhand • Nagpur • Patna • Pune • Uttarakhand

Disclaimer

Science and technology are constantly changing fields. New research and experience broaden the scope of information and knowledge. The author had tried his best in giving information available to him while preparing the material for this book. Although all efforts has been made to ensure optimum accuracy of the material, yet it is quite possible some errors might have been left uncorrected. The publisher, the printer and the author will not be held responsible for any inadvertent errors or inaccuracies.

AETCOM

Attitude, EThics and COMmunication

MANUAL

Learning Modules for MBBS Professional Year II

Competencies for the Indian Medical Graduate

As Recommended by National Medical Commission

ISBN: 978-93-5466-626-1

First Edition: 2024

Reprint: **2026**

Published by **Satish Kumar Jain** and produced by **Varun Jain** for

CBS Publishers & Distributors Pvt Ltd

4819/XI Prahlad Street, 24 Ansari Road, Daryaganj, New Delhi 110 002, India
Ph: 011-23266838, 23289259 Website: www.cbspd.com
e-mail: delhi@cbspd.com

Corporate Office: 204 FIE, Industrial Area, Patparganj, Delhi 110 092, India
Ph: 011-49344934 Fax: 011-49344935 e-mail: publishing@cbspd.com; publicity@cbspd.com

Branches

- **Bengaluru:** Seema House 2975, 17th Cross, K.R. Road, Banasankari 2nd Stage Bengaluru 560 070, Karnataka, India
  Ph: +91-80-26771678/79 Fax: +91-80-26771680 e-mail: bangalore@cbspd.com
- **Chennai:** 18/8B, Subbarayan Street, Shenoy Nagar, Chennai 600 030, Tamil Nadu, India
  Ph: +91-44-42032115, 45022115 e-mail: chennai@cbspd.com
- **Kochi:** 42/1325, 1326, Power House Road, Opposite KSEB, Power House, Kochi, 682018 Kerala, India
  Ph: +91-484-4059061–65 Fax: +91-484-4059065 e-mail: kochi@cbspd.com
- **Kolkata:** 147, Hind Ceramics Compound, 1st Floor, Nilgunj Road, Belghoria, Kolkata 700056 West Bengal, India
  Ph: +91-33-25633055/56 e-mail: kolkata@cbspd.com
- **Lucknow:** Basement, Khushnuma Complex, 7 Meerabai Marg (behind Jawahwar Bhawan) Lucknow 226001, UP, India
  Ph: +91-522-4000032 e-mail: tiwari.lucknow@cbspd.com
- **Mumbai:** PWD Shed, Gala No. 25/26, Ramchandra Bhatt Marg, Next JJ Hospital, Gate No. 2 Opp. Union Bank of India, Noorbaug Mumbai 400009, Maharashtra, India
  Ph: +91-22-66661880/89 e-mail: mumbai@cbspd.com

Representatives

- **Gujarat** • **Hyderabad** • **Jharkhand** • **Nagpur** • **Patna** • **Pune** • **Uttarakhand**

For trade terms please contact customercare@cbspd.com
For general enquiries please contact info@cbspd.com

Printed at: Mudrak, Noida, UP, India

Preface

It gives me immense pleasure to present *AETCOM* for Second MBBS Professional. I would like to emphasize that introduction of course on Attitude, Ethics and Communication as Learning Modules for MBBS student was one of the very important milestones in medical education as recommended by National Medical Commission. The medical students have to achieve professional expertise and to become competent doctors. It is not only the knowledge and competency which is required but a medical student's needs to be groomed to achieve clinical and communication skills as well. The book has been designed to inculcate high moral principle and ethical values. This book covers the curriculum and syllabus designed for students of MBBS as per recommendation of National Medical Commission. The book also covers important topics on medical ethics as recommended by Medical Councils of various South Asian countries, UK, US, Canada, New Zealand and Australia. The key features of the book are that it has simplified text for easy reproducibility, it has well defined learning objectives at beginning of each chapter, it is written in easy, lucid and comprehensive language and it includes case scenarios for interactive learning and for better grasping of concepts. The manual is so designed that student can note lecture points; resolve case scenarios, write formative and summative assessment; and moreover after completion of the course a record is available to evaluate students performance and grade them.

I am thankful to Dr Vikas Bhatia, Director, All India Institute of Medical Sciences, Bibinagar, Hyderabad, for his encouragement and support. I am thankful to Mr Satish Jain (CMD) and Mr YN Arjuna (Senior Vice President—Publishing, Editorial and Publicity), CBS Publishers & Distributors Pvt Ltd and all publishing staff.

I am thankful to my mother Mrs Ujwala Parekh, wife Dr Jyoti and son Joshua for all their support in this endeavor.

I hope that the book will stand immensely helpful to all the readers. All efforts have been made to write the script in flawless manner, and mistakes, if any, due to oversight may be pardoned. Looking forward for your suggestions to come up with the next edition based on your feedback.

Nitin Ashok John

Contents

Index of Competencies

Competency based Undergraduate Curriculum for the Indian Medical Graduate

Module

2.1

The Foundations of Communication

Learning Objectives: The students at end of lecture should be able to demonstrate the ability to communicate to patients in a patient, respectful, non-threatening, non-judgmental and empathetic manner. The role play/case study discussed in the chapter are self- designed for giving insight regarding the topic. The teacher can formulate case study from practical experience or live situation in their setup for teaching concepts to the students.

SESSION I

Introductory Small Group Session (1 hour)

Key Points

1. Communication is a key skill required to be imbibed by medical students for effective health care management.
2. Recording patient history is an art. The medical student's needs to maintain calm and patience enough listening to patients complain carefully and noting it meticulously.
3. Medical students must address their patients with due respect in non-threatening and non-judgmental manner.
4. The genuine concern for addressing patients suffering and their health need should be the primary goal.
5. The patient's literacy level should also be considered while recording their medical illness history as illiterate patient may not be able to express health issues properly.
6. The essential qualities that will help medical students in developing clinical communication skills are patient listening, genuine concern for patient's agony and health issues, and their impetus and readiness to acquire the needed skills.

7. With effective communication the medical student can develop a good rapport with patients, understand patients health issue better, allay patients fears and worries and eventually build the patients confidence and trust.

Thus, to conclude the communication is basic pillar of strength in providing effective health care services.

Purpose for Communication

The main purpose for communication in hospital setting is for:

1. Eliciting and recording the clinical history of patients.
2. Discussing with patients their health status and management strategies.
3. To health educate and counsel patients.
4. Developing rapport with the patients.
5. Build patients trust and confidence.
6. Getting feedback during follow-up from patients after treatment.
7. Solving any queries of patients.

The important modes of communication include:

1. **Oral communication**
2. **Written communication**

Communication and Challenging Occasions to be addressed in hospital setup includes:

1. Delivering sad news such as death of patient or to patient's relative.
2. Informing regarding critical state of patient to patient or patient's relative.
3. Communication with patient who is upset or to anxious patient's relative in OPD / IPD.
4. Informing regarding treatment strategies and cost of treatment to the poor patients.
5. Communication with patients having impaired hearing.
6. Communicating after receiving negative feedback regarding the treatment which was given; from patients or patient's relative.

CONCLUSION

The respectful, non-judgmental non-threatening and empathetic communication of doctors with patient is the most vital aspects of effective health care delivery to the patients.

BIBLIOGRAPHY

1. Bowman D, Cushing A. Ethics, law and communication. In: Kumar P, Clark M, (Eds). Kumar and Clarke's Clinical Medicine, 9th ed. Philadelphia, PA: Elsevier; 2017:chap 1.
2. Bukstein DA. Patient adherence and effective communication. Ann Allergy Asthma Immunol. 2016;117(6):613–9.
3. Crozier WR. Blushing and the Social Emotions: The Self Unmasked (New York: Palgrave Macmillan, 2006).
4. Emotional Intelligence and its Impact on Communication in the Workplacehttps://franchetti.com/emotionalintelligence-impact-communication-workplace/ October 11, 2016.
5. Evans D Emotion: The Science of Sentiment (New York: Oxford University Press, 2001:5–6.
6. Gilligan T, Coyle N, Frankel RM, et al. Patient clinician communication: American Society of Clinical Oncology consensus guideline. J Clin Oncol. 2017;35(31):3618–32.
7. Hashim MJ. Patient-Centered Communication: Basic Skills. Am Fam Physician. 2017 Jan 1;95(1):29–34.
8. Hausberg M. Enhancing medical students' communication skills: development and evaluation of an undergraduate training program. BMC Medical Education 2012;12:16.
9. Kotchemidova C. "Emotion Culture and Cognitive Constructions of Reality," Communication Quarterly 2010;58(2):207–34.
10. LaNoue MD, Roter DL. Exploring patient centeredness: The relationship between self-reported empathy and patient-centered communication in medical trainees. Patient Educ Couns. 2018 Jun; 101(6):1143–1146.
11. Makoul G. Essential elements of communication in medical encounters: the Kalamazoo consensus statement. Acad Med. 2001, Apr; 76(4):390–3.
12. Mehta A, Adams N, Fredrickson M, Kraszkiewicz W, Siy J, Hamel L, Hendel Paterson B. Craving Empathy: Studying the Sustained Impact of Empathy Training on Clinicians. J Patient Exp. 2021 Sep. 27;8: 23743735211043383.
13. Nitin Ashok John, Jyoti Elgiva John. Effective Communication Skills Facilitates Better Health Care Delivery. Br J Pharm Med Res, 2022;7(1):3527–32.
14. Peters, John Durham. Speaking into the air: a history of the idea of communication. Chicago: University of Chicago Press, 1999;2.
15. Rime B. "Interpersonal Emotion Regulation," in Handbook of Emotion Regulation, James J (Ed.), Gross, New York: Guilford Press, 2007:466–8.
16. Salovey P, Alison Woolery, John D. Mayer, "Emotional Intelligence: Conceptualization and Measurement," in Blackwell Handbook of Social Psychology: Interpersonal Processes, Garth JO Fletcher and Margaret S Clark, Malden MA (Eds.): Blackwell, 2011:279–307.

SESSION II

Focused Small Group Session (2 hours)

Goal: Focused small group session with role play where the students have an opportunity to observe, criticize and discuss common mistakes in opening the discussion, listening and data gathering.

Activity

1. The students are divided among groups with 10 student members in each group.
2. The students are told to enact a role play in reference to goal mentioned as above with doctor addressing a patient.
3. An alternate group of 10 students will observe the role play and students shall observe, criticize and discuss common mistakes in opening the discussion, listening and data gathering.

Note: Both group will enact a role play alternatively and so also comment on ideal situations and criticism of role play.

Role Play 1 (Participant Group 1: Ex Roll Nos 1–10)

Mimicked Venue: Banjara Hills Nursing Home

Place: Visitors room outside the consultant room where receptionist is busy receiving appointment call:

Renuka **(Receptionist)**: Yes Madam, noted your name ... You are waiting No. 31 … Now checkup of patient No. 14 is in progress.

Meanwhile in waiting room:

Ravi **(Patient No. 15) to Receptionist:** Madam I am ready with reports to go in ...

Suddenly **Mrs Shanti steps in** with mother ...

Renuka **(Receptionist):** Ignoring patient No. 15 ... Renuka … exclaims ... Hello Shanti … seeing you after long time.

Shanti Oh Renuka … Are you working here? You were my obedient student while you were studying in school … Well … Renuka ... Please take my son inside ... to doctor as he is having fever ...

Renuka **(Receptionist):** Sure Madam … Come

Ravi **(Patient No. 15) to Receptionist:** But ... its my turn now

Renuka **(Receptionist):** Come on Mr Anil ... Don't fuss … Please wait

Renuka **(Receptionist) to Dr Gaddam:** Sir she is my friend Shanti, her son is not well …

Dr Gaddam Please come in … Have a seat …

Ramu **(Patient: Shanti's Son):** Sat on examination stool

Dr Gaddam What's your name?

Ramu

Dr Gaddam Well I hope all fine Ramu … But you look to be sick

Ramu Doctor having fever with chilled feeling since morning …

Dr Gaddam Any vomiting, loose motions, fatigue ...

Ramu Just having body ache

Dr Gaddam Well any past history of any epilepsy: I mean fits, or chronic illness

Ramu No. Sir

Dr Gaddam Any addiction to tobacco or alcohol

Ramu No. sir … never

Dr Gaddam Doctors makes detail general and physical examination after instructing Ramu to lie on the Couch.

Dr Gaddam Records all clinical history and details and write medication and explains it to Shanti and Ramu

Dr Gaddam later: You will be well soon Ramu ...

Visit after 5 days for review ...

Nurse Vishaka who is assisting Dr Gaddam accompanies patient outward

Ravi (Patient No. 15) to Receptionist as she instructs to go inside … You have wasted my time … How can you send patient coming later before me … Renuka Snubs

Ravi (Patient No. 15) to Dr Gaddam: Doctor your receptionist was partial...

Dr Gaddam Please stop your unnecessary arguments … Yes what are your health related complaints

Ravi Doctor pain in abdomen and loose motions since yesterday night ... and

Dr Gaddam Ok ... Ok ... He writes the prescription and ask him to go

Ravi Sir—how to take these medicines …

Dr Gaddam Well Chemist will tell you … Bye

Observation by (Participant Group 11: Ex Roll Nos 11–20)

An alternate group of 10 students to observe the role play and observe, criticize and discuss common mistakes in opening the discussion, listening and data gathering.

The students shall discuss and record their opinion below:

The Group teacher / Facilitator to make opinion regarding student's presentation: The students to note important clues and corrective action below: Ideal situational modification in such scenario:

Role Play 2 (Participant Group 11: Ex Roll Nos 11–20)

Dr Vivek(**ENT Surgeon**): Sister … **Sister Sara** … Where are you?

SaraWell Sir … Coming ... Tell me Sir

Dr VivekSee I am busy with attending webnair today … see to it … that patients are send faster in ... Record their preliminary complaints ... I may not be able to spend enough time on them ...

Sara Sir I am working with you for last 15 years and know management regime too ... if you say—I will write that too ...

Dr VivekWell you can do it in simpler cases ... ok ... well can leave it to me too ...

See that receptionist Vijay collect the fees from patients ... prior only … my consultation fees I mean

Dr VivekYes, come in

Dinkar**(Patient):** Sir I am having sneezing since ... tring ... tring ... Dr Vivek's phone is ringing ... his wife on line ...

Dr Vivek Yes, Preeti ... tell me ... well Dinkar continue ... yes, sneezing and ... Ok Preeti I will come home soon …

Dr VivekDinkar: Take these medicine

DinkarBut Sir I have sore throat ...

Dr Vivek... Well all Viral ... Go

Dr VivekNext patient

RajiniDoctor I have headache, giddiness, etc.

Dr Vivek is on his blue tooth—ok ok ok ... Rajini—take these medicines …

Rajinihow many days...

Dr VivekCome on I am busy ... Ask nurse

Dr Vivek Nurse ... see to it all complaints are recorded by you only—you know, I am busy and these patients... Oh My...

Observation by (Participant Group 1: Ex Roll Nos 1–10)

An alternate group of 10 students to observe the role play and observe, criticize and discuss common mistakes in opening the discussion, listening and data gathering.

The students shall discuss and record their opinion below:

The Group teacher / Facilitator to make opinion regarding student's presentation: The students to note important clues and corrective action below: Ideal situational modification in such scenario:

Exercise 1

Students are instructed to go through the paper and describe the importance of communication in effective health care delivery and record their findings here

Link–Paper... Hashim MJ. Patient–Centered Communication: Basic Skills. Am Fam Physician. 2017 Jan 1;95(1):29–34.

SESSION III

Skills lab sessions where students can perform tasks on standardized or regular patients with opportunity for self critique, critique by patient and by the facilitator.

Exercise 1: Explaining treatment regime to patient

1. Ask students in small group to enact on mannequin method of self injecting insulin to a patient of insulin-dependent diabetes mellitus.
2. Then advice regarding the other medicines to be taken.
3. Advice of do's and don'ts as safety measures to prevent hypoglycemia in patients of diabetes.
4. Follow-up advice

Point of inaction during above role play

1. One participant each will be doctor, nurse, patient, nursing attendant and two patients relatives (Two students to direct the role play and Two students to play role of self critique)
2. One facilitator to overall coordinate, guide and opine.

The students to write the complete enacted role story, opinion as self critique, patient's critique comments and facilitator comments below:

Exercise 2

Communicating and recording a case history of patient of Asthma/ Diabetes/Hypertension, etc.

Action: Small Group Task

1. Two student to records patients illness history as doctor.
2. Two observer students can be self critique who shall assess the pitfall in effective communication.

3. Two observer students to interact with patients in effective, empathetic, non-judgmental and non threatening way to record patients history.
4. Facilitator to opine and conclude the sessions.

The students to write the enacted interaction, opinion of self critique, patient's critique comments and facilitator comments below:

Students Assessment by Faculty In-charge

1. **Formative:** Participation in session II and participation in session III may be used as part of formative assessment.

Name of Student: ....

Participation in session II:
Excellent/Very Good/Good/Satisfactory/Poor

Signature: Faculty In-charge, AETCOM ....

Participation in session III:
Excellent/Very Good/Good/Satisfactory/Poor

Signature: Faculty In-charge, AETCOM ....

2. Summative: May be deferred.

Viva Voce or written exams of 20 marks:

Questions

1. **Why effective communication skills are required in medical practice?**

A.

2. **Define communication, its purpose and modes of communication.**

A.

3. Describe the various modes of communication.

A.

4. Describe the communication process.

A.

5. Describe the modalities of effective patient centric communication.

A.

6. Describe communication and challenging occasions to be addressed in hospital setup.

A.

7. Describe the communication skills you learned from the chapter.

A.

Module

2.2

The Foundations of Bioethics

Learning Objectives: The student should be able to understand and discuss:

1. Role of nonmaleficence as a guiding principle in patient care.
2. Role of autonomy and shared responsibility as a guiding principle in patient care.
3. Role of beneficence of a guiding principle in patient care.
4. Role of a physician in health care system.
5. Role of justice as a guiding principle in patient.

Lecture Session (2 hours)

Introduction

The four important principles of bioethics are beneficence, autonomy nonmaleficence and justice. These fundamental principles form the strong pillars of bioethics as they are implicated as part of good clinical practice. These foursome principles immensely help health care professionals in making rightful decisive judgment while addressing arising moral issues at work place in a hospital setup. Irrespective of an individual's own ideologies and philosophy; there is less likely that any issues can arise for effective health care delivery by physicians as these four prima facie principles are binding and are rightly fitted in out frame of moral responsibilities in health care delivery.

Discussion

Role of nonmaleficence as a guiding principle in patient care.

Nonmaleficence

Background: The health care professionals are strongly bonded to the ethical medical practices as they pledge to follow stringently the directive of medical law and ethics prevailing in the country. Caring and treating the patients using all the best clinical acumen and judgment by physician which he/she possesses is the corner stone of medical practice. Moreover doing no harm is the most vital principle in good clinical practice which a physician abides too irrespective even if the patient has requested this for.

Considering the moral sense of duties and responsibilities towards patients the dotor provides the best medical care.

Definition

Nonmaleficence is a word which has been derived from the ancient maxim primum non nocere, and is translated from Latin original language as first, do no harm.

Principle of Nonmaleficence

The nonmaleficence principle instructs physicians to "do no harm" towards the patients irrespective of their act of commission or omission. They are expected to refrain from prescribing ineffective treatments and manifest no malice or ill feeling towards the patients. But the two sides of the same sword there are beneficial effect of drug therapy as well as potential risks of side effects and adverse events but addressing the associated ethical issues it is necessary that the physician forsee the benefits outweighing the harms.

The physicians should not provide any treatment protocol which will pose risk for patients rather than any benefits as this would harm the patients.

Moreover a physician is expected to provide a standard health care expected to being provided by a competent doctor and ensure that they should be no harm or in situation minimal risk which can be justified under moral convictions; as well as those tenable under medical law and ethics. This principle affirms the need for medical competence. Physician may make mistakes in management by act of omission but medical negligence is not warranted for.

Exceptions

1. **Scenario in which a physician has to decide when harm seems inevitable:** A pregnant lady having developed uterine carcinoma while doctor who is bound to act under principle of nonmaleficence is under dilemma is whether to save mother by performing hysterectomy and scarifying baby.

   In such situation when act of morality against act of duty is foreseen the patient has the right to decide regarding her fate as act of self-defense to accept hysterectomy for saving her own life and/or accept or avoid the unintentional and undesired outcome of death of her fetus. The patient consent and decision has a final say doctor should discuss and inform patient regarding the most recent and reliable evidence-based information and knowledge in order to permit patient to take a conscious decision on further line of management.

2. **Potential harm by drugs:** The medical and pharmacological decisions carry the potential for harm due to adverse and side effects of every drug molecule, but harm is to be overweighed by physician against the feasible health benefits.

3. **Exceptional situational shift in principle of nonmaleficence in individuals practicing potentially harmful behaviours:** The community health care practices where degrees of harm are weighed over likely chances of occurrence of greater harms or plausible health benefits. This can be cited with an example such as imposition of prohibition of smoking in public areas may have a direct harm and negative impact in terms of mental health in addicted smokers but at the same time it will prevent the community members from harmful effect of passive smoking as this would have cause greater damage in public with large number of individuals being exposed to passive smoke in the community. The intricacy in such tricky situation is that either away imposition of prohibition over smoking is preventing further harm against their pulmonary health of smokers as well as preventing lung damage in community by passive effect of cigarette smoke.

Conclusively the principle of nonmaleficence articulates a fundamental commitment of causing no harm to the patient.

Role of Autonomy and Shared Responsibility as a Guiding Principle in Patient Care

Respect for Autonomy

In medical health care it is important that the doctor shares the information about the patient's health with the patient as patients management is a joint responsibility in which physician has to provide standard health care and in process obtained consent regarding proposed treatment, surgery, therapy, etc. and plausible side effects and adverse events if any associated with the management. In case of minor, mentally insane or very old geriatric patients having cognition issues consent of parents, guardians and relatives is must. The patients voluntary participation in decision making is must. The patient must consent with understanding with her/ his own will and must not act under any pressure or influence in decision-making.

Example: The patients may be left to make their decision of excepting management and treatment for their diseases and especially can make decisions under the principle of autonomy as per their liking, loyalty, religious beliefs, life values and moral principles. The doctors are encountered with patients who do not believe in accepting a blood transfusion. The physician should make the patient aware of the life threats of refusing blood transfusion, but under principle of autonomy the patient can decide over excepting blood transfusion over death or vice versa. The communication even then by physician should be with compassion, respect, nonthreatening and non judgmental even if the views are differing from the standard goals of medical management practice. Physician should explain harm over benefit the best of their approach capabilities. Howsoever, some physicians differ in such a situation and harp that the principle of nonmaleficence also needed to be taken into consideration and recommend that such a case needs interpretation in light of the patient's belief system about the nature of harms.

An emergency situation when patient is unconscious and if parents/guardians are explained the risk over gain usually the relatives prefer to follow doctors instruction. The physician must obtain written consent in such a situation.

Role of Beneficence of a Guiding Principle in Patient Care

1. **Definition:** Beneficence is a principle under medical ethics which states that the physicians should provide standard health care to patients to the best of his / her ability and should ensure good health benefits and cause no harm to the patients.
2. **Principle of Beneficence:** The physician should provided standard health care in the best interest of the patient. It is an act of being kind so as to bring about a positive outcome in patients health and should ensure good health benefits and cause no harm to the patients.

   The principle of beneficence encompasses certain moral rules or obligations which includes:
   - Protecting and defending the rights of others.
   - Preventing from occurring harm to others.
   - Removing conditions which may cause harm to others.
   - Helping individual who are physically challenged.
   - Rescuing individuals who are in danger.
3. Beneficence is a primary ethical principle which ensures promotion and protection of the patient's wellbeing in complete patient's interests.
4. Beneficence harness on principle of relieving the causative symptoms impairing the quality of life in case of a person who is dying.
5. Beneficence ensures that physician consider individual circumstances and recalls and ascertains that what was good for a patient may not be necessarily good or beneficial for another.

To conclude beneficence is as an act of kindness, charity and mercy with a intention of doing good to others under aegis of moral obligation.

Role of a Physician in Health Care System

The physicians are medically qualified doctors who examine patients, diagnose and treat them. Moreover, they actively participate in health educating their patients and patient's relatives, play active role in implementing national health care programs and ensure preventive measures to prevent spread of any communicable diseases or infections especially in time of epidemics.

The physician being multifaceted plays many vital roles while discharging duties as health care provider and these are:

1. **Role as team leader:** The physicians are team leader in hospital setup and play active role in coordinating, directing, communicating, supervising for imparting effective health care delivery.
2. **Treatment and management of disease:** The physician treats and manage the disease in patients as this is their primary duties.
3. **Catering heath delivery:** Physician caters their services at various health centers and these may be primary health centers at village level, secondary health care (at district level hospitals) and tertiary health care (medical colleges and health institute of national importance and higher learning, etc.) settings.
4. **Role in health education:** The physicians also health educates, their team of paramedics, nurses, technicians, multipurpose workers, etc., while managing patients which also help in improving the clinical skills of paramedics.
5. **Role in health economics and as a social entrepreneur:** The physician plans health care delivery in an appropriate, cost-effective manner in concurrence with the national health care policies. This helps to establish economically viable health care delivery preventing any financial wastage and losses.
6. **Role in generating health care data:** The physician prescribes various investigations for patients and manages patients aiding in their faster recovery. This data generated over the years of investigative findings and management strategies can be analyzed and opined for planning future management strategies.
7. **Role in prevention of diseases:** Physicians advice preventive measure strategies to prevent spreading of communicable diseases in the community. Similarly, they promote and recommend lifestyle changes in patients of obesity, diabetes, hypertension, thyroid disease, etc.
8. **Role in improving quality of life and lifespan:** The physician provides therapeutic, curative, preventive and rehabilitative health care services thereby reducing health burden in community and thus eventually improving human quality of life and lifespan of patients.
9. **Role in management of epidemics:** Physician helps in reducing risk of catastrophic situations as in epidemics by timely intervention and management.

10. **Role as a behavioural therapist in community:** The physician practicing with humanistic approach (treating with compassion and care) helps building trust of patients and this has found to be effective in developing confidence, solace and optimistic hope in patient thereby hastening recovery.
11. **Role in building professionalism and respect towards doctor community:** The professionalism in practices by doctors such as abiding by codes of ethics establishes high ethical standards and this helps in looking forwards towards doctors with respect, trust and confidence by community members thus establishing medical profession at high esteem in the community.
12. **Role as trainers of present and future generation of doctors for community:** The physicians provide on job training in teaching as well as service hospitals thus are developing man force for future health care delivery. This also helps in improving the standard of patient care.
13. **Role as authoritative sources on clinical standards:** The physicians continue lifelong learning to update their medical knowledge thus they are looked forward as authoritative sources on clinical standards and practice for diagnosis and management by the community members for seeking consultation if required.
14. **Participation in national health care program:** The physician participates in implementing various national health care programs in community such as family welfare program, national tuberculosis management program, national program for prevention of malaria, leprosy, tuberculosis, etc.
15. **Participating as social workers:** The physician especially provides honorary services in shelter homes, home for the aged, slums, prison, or as a health provider NGO, etc. and thus provides social service to the community.
16. **Role in changing dynamics of the patient health care:** The advancement in scientific technology and innovations (example: telemedicine and employing artificial intelligence) makes it essential for physicians to upgrade to understand and imbibe the changed dynamics of the patient health care and its delivery.
17. **Provides services matching local area health care needs:** The physicians also must match the local area health care needs depending on the disease prevalent in those areas, innovation in machinery methodology of investigative protocols and modified treatment regime of diseases, and state and nations legislative initiatives (applicable laws, Consumer Protection Act).

Role of Justice as a Guiding Principle in Patient

Principle of Justice

Justice as a term is a form of fairness more specifically it is giving to each what is their due.

The characteristic components in discharge of justice in health care system include:

1. The distribution of health resources to be fair and equitable for each individuals of the community. Under principle of justice, there is need for promoting the sustainable health system for the larger good of society.
2. In case when resources such as medicines are scarce, fair means of allocating such scarce resources needs to be planned so that the most needy receive the benefit first, though every individual is entitled for equal treatment; all efforts should be made my health care providers to resolve scarcity issues. Government should provide adequate resources in terms of manpower, equipment and medicines, etc. to help overcome the crisis situation.
3. The criteria for distributive justice are based on various facts and criterion which include:
   - Equal share for each individual
   - Allocation to every individual according to need
   - Allocation to every individual according to his/her effort
   - Allocation to every individual according to their contribution
   - Allocation to every individual according to merit.

   But the fact under justice which needs to prevail is equal allocation to every individual according to the need.
4. The needs of the entire population should be taken into account while planning for future health care delivery strategies so that with equity all resources are accessible to all in population.
5. Health inequalities are unwarranted, unfair and totally unjust.
6. Under uniform principle of justice it is necessary that no individual are discriminated and excluded for any planned intervention, all act in planned intervention should be transparent, no individual is exposed to any risk in any planned intervention and all planned strategies should refrain from damaging the sense of social cohesion and solidarity.

BIBLIOGRAPHY

1. Beauchamp T, Childress J. Principles of Biomedical Ethics, 7th Edition. New York: Oxford University Press, 2013.
2. Beauchamp TL, Childress JF. Principles of Biomedical Ethics. New York: Oxford University Press; 2009.
3. Bolhuis S. Toward process-oriented teaching for self-directed lifelong learning: a multidimensional perspective. Learning Instruction 2003; 13:327–47.
4. Daniels N. Just Health: Meeting Health Needs Fairly. 2008, Cambridge: Cambridge University Press.
5. Davis DA, Thomson MA, Oxman AD, Haynes RB. Changing physician performance. A systematic review of the effect of continuing medical education strategies. JAMA 1995;274:700–5.
6. Frankena, WK. Ethics, 2nd Edition. Englewood Cliffs, NJ: Prentice-Hall, 1973.
7. Gert B, Culver CM, Clouser KD. Bioethics a Return to Fundamentals. New York: Oxford University Press, 1997.
8. Gillon R. Medical ethics: four principles plus attention to scope. BMJ. 1994 Jul 16;309(6948):184–8.
9. Hippocrates. The history of epidemics. Samuel Farr (trans.) London: T. Cadell, 1780.
10. Hojat M, Gonnella JS, Erdmann JB, Veloski JJ, Xu G. Primary care and non-primary care physicians: a longitudinal study of their similarities. Acad Med 1995;70:S17–28.
11. Jonsen A, Siegler M, Winslade W. Ethics, 7th Edition. New York: McGraw-Hill Medical, 2010.
12. Jonsen AR. Do no harm: axiom of medical ethics. In: Spicker SF, Englehardt HT (Jr), editors. Philosophical Medical Ethics: Its Nature and Significance. Dordrecht, the Netherlands: Springer; 1977. pp. 27–41.
13. Mazmanian PE, Davis DA. Continuing medical education and the physician as a learner: guide to the evidence. JAMA 2002;288:1057–60.
14. McCormick, TR. Ethical issues inherent to Jehovah's Witnesses. Perioperative Nursing Clinics 2008;3(3):253–9.
15. Principles of Bioethics, Author: Thomas R. McCormick, D. Min., Senior Lecturer Emeritus, Dept. Bioethics and Humanities, School of Medicine, University of Washington.
16. Rawls J. A Theory of Justice. Cambridge, MA: Harvard University Press, 1999.
17. Schröder-Bäck P, Duncan P, Sherlaw W, Brall C, Czabanowska K. Teaching seven principles for public health ethics: towards a curriculum for a short course on ethics in public health programmes. BMC Med Ethics 2014 Oct 7;15:73.

18. Skrzypczyk-Ostaszewicz A, Rubach M. Gynaecological cancers coexisting with pregnancy—a literature review. Contemp Oncol (Pozn) 2016;20(3):193–8.
19. Smith CM. Origin and uses of primum non-nocere—above all, do no harm! J Clin Pharmacol 2005;45:371–7.

Disclaimer: All information in chapter **(Module 2.2)** The Foundations of Bioethics includes but not limited to; and is for information purpose only. The author declares that the sincere attempt has been made to give standard accurate information in the chapter, but it is not a substitute for any legal or professional advice. The reader should seek advice from legal professional if they are seek consultation and advice for any issue associated with foundation of bioethics.

ASSIGNMENT

Summative:

The students after reading the chapter should write short notes on

(a) Autonomy

(b) Beneficence

(c) Nonmaleficence

Module

2.3

Health Care as a Right

Learning Objectives: The students at end of lecture should be able to understand and discuss:

1. Role of justice as a guiding principle in patient care.
2. If health care as a right?
3. Implications of health care as a right?
4. Social and economic implications of health care as a right?
5. Missing links and the implications for doctors?

HEALTH CARE AS A RIGHT

Teaching Protocol: A lecture-cum-seminar of 2 hours duration in which students are exposed to topic and supplemented with references material for reading and students in groups can present seminar with conclusive discussion by the teacher.

Background: The students to be introduced to health care systems, access health care to all, principle of equity of access, impact of socio-economic situations detrimental to health care access and the role of the physician in the health care system.

Discussion

Justice as a guiding principle in patient care

Key Points

1. Justice in health care system refers that each individual of the community shall have a fair, equitable, and appropriate access to health care.
2. More relevant reference in health care system is the distributive justice which refers to fair and equitable distribution of health care resources.

3. Principle of justice under distribution of health care resources: Every individual of community must receive an equal share of health resources, as per their need, as per the effort and contribution, as per merit, and according to free-market exchanges.
4. The above principles cannot be a fit protocol at all times and needs a balancing act of considering few or all principle for workable solution while distributing medical resources.
5. Current initiative under Government of India includes such as AYUSHMAN Scheme Bharat Yojana (National Digital Health Policy) which is providing health insurance to the poor.
6. Under principle of justice equal time for examination of each patient should be done by physician but it is not possible under every situation as patients disease may be mild infection or acute or chronic condition.
7. **Dilemmas in Justice:**
   A. Physician primarily should be fair while prescribing medicines to patients and not expensive drugs for rich and cheaper drugs for poor but must ensure that the best effective drug to be given suiting the disease condition. Moreover, generally free drug supply is available for poor people under various welfare schemes run by the **central government** and state government.
   B. Prioritizing treatment for cancer patient is must for their survival but its debated that other chronic illnesses cannot be just overruled for benefit of one as by doing so we limit other patients to access health care.

Note: Justice as part of ethics discussion can be argued among group if whether the physician acts in situation of dilemma affects ones human rights? Whether the action priority is partial towards one group over other group?

HEALTH CARE AS A RIGHT

Key Points

1. Every human has a right to access health care delivery provided by the state under right to confidentiality, right of being informed regarding his/her health condition, right to life and right to receive quality health care without any discrimination due to his caste, creed, sex, race, religion and financial condition.
2. Fundamental right to health as practiced in many countries include right to receive appropriate health care and humane treatment, right to choose the health care provider of their own choice and right to be informed regarding their state of condition, planned diagnostic and therapeutic protocol and further line of management.
3. **Scenario in India:** The Constitution of India does not expressly recognizes a fundamental right to health but the right of life in Constitution of India has

been cohesively expressed as part of right to life under article 21. But the constitution does mention it in reference to public health specifying states role and responsibility in providing health care to its population.

Few Examples: The state under directive principles of State Policy as per provision in Part IV of Constitution of India which specifies the basis for the right to health for the public. The directive has been laid for the state to secure health of workers under Article 39(E) of Constitution of India. Article 41 of Constitution of India has laid public ordinances for health care of old aged, sick and disabled persons to the states.

Article 42 of Constitution of India has laid directive for the state to offer just and humane conditions of work and provisions for maternity relief. The Article 47 of Constitution of India directs state to raise level of minimum standard of life for improving public health.

Constitution of India directs states to enhance public health care facilities and also ask them to ensure that the municipalities and panchayats strengthen public health under Article 243G. A legislatively guaranteed right for health in India; will definitely make fair, just and equitable access to health care a legally binding and ensure accountability.

4. **Conclusion:** The right to health care implies a individual right for safe-guarding his health from any hazardous action of state and but state is obligated to provide health care at an affordable price.
5. Current initiative under Government of India includes under the AYUSHMAN Scheme Bharat Yojana (National Digital Health Policy) which is providing health insurance to the poor.
6. The state government apart from its role in delivering effective primary health care must also ensure that the other determinants of health, as safe and potable drinking water, sanitation in community, nutritive food consumption, housing facilities, health education, and gender equality are safe-guarded for the public.
7. Involvement of non-governmental organizations in effective health care delivery must be meaningful in terms of its active involvement in various phases of programming: assessment, analysis, planning, implementation, monitoring and evaluation.
8. Under provision of health care as fundamental right; health care facilities, goods that are medicines, and services must be accessible to all in community with no discrimination with easy physical, economical and information accessibility.

IMPLICATIONS OF HEALTH CARE AS A RIGHT

Key Points

Health care as right for citizen is a must desired provision to be provided by any country for its citizens.

1. **Need for addressing to growing health care needs:** The primary implications of health care as a right is the addressing the health care needs of growing world population. As effective health care delivery will need more hospitals, more manpower, more equipment, and more medicine for increasing population. Matching supply demand need is challenging. The challenges are that how to balance the financial investment on health care program.
2. **Addressing issues regarding increased prevalence of diseases:** Increasing morbidity due to diseases in developing country and cancers in advance economy countries due to ever-changing lifestyle and food habits the incidences of new cases of noncommunicable diseases (NCDs) such as obesity, metabolic syndrome, diabetes, hypertension is rising globally and is a challenge as implications of appropriate health care for all.
3. **Need for developing model doctor–patient relationship approach:** The medical professionals who provide health care are under moral obligation to extend respectful approach towards patients respecting their dignity and autonomy of patients. In this regard there will be need to define a well planned protocol of legal and ethical standards of behavioural approach while treating patients but challenge posed towards it is that it may not match with temperament and informed choices of the individual patient. Eventually, it may land up with doctors being concerned in understanding mental temperament apart from delivering standard medical care especially in condition when health care is defined under category of fundamental rights. Hence, counseling of patients for understanding standard medical care in their situation may help handling the situation.
4. **Financial implication on Government Budget:** Approach of government towards providing adequate health resources for all is itself a challenge in implication of health care as fundamental rights. In India, government has been allocating adequate funds for strengthening the public health infrastructures such as building more hospitals; employ more doctors and paramedics as part of fulfilling increased need of human resource, effective supply chain management of drugs to government hospitals and centers, setting new medical colleges for robust medical education system as this will create more workforce; and so also government be ensuring acts and regulation of private health care providers through legislative enforcement for an accountable health care delivery.
5. **Social status of patient and its relation to health as fundamental right:**
   A. If people in community are illiterate; they may not understand the need and importance of treating diseases with modern medicine. They may refuse to take treatment or may not be willing to come for follow up. An educated person may understand and utilize his fundamental rights better.
   B. An educated person will have good job and can access health care facilities provided by government as mostly those working in government set up are insured with Central Government Health Scheme, Employees State Insurance Scheme, AYUSHMAN Bharat Health Scheme, etc.

Employed individuals can make better choices about education, child care, food, shelter, health care, etc. Good housing, clean surrounding, consumption of healthy food and seeking medical care during illness are the chain followed by financially well sustained family.

C. Better social connects are fundamentally helping in people being healthy as they have better mental frame of mind as well as they may get easy information regarding health schemes from their social network.

SOCIAL AND ECONOMICAL IMPLICATIONS OF HEALTH CARE AS RIGHT

Key Points

1. The social determinants of health, influencing health equity in positivity or negativity are: Employment, income, social protection, and education level, life conditions at work place, food, housing, early childhood maturity and development and social connect affect how healthy and how long we live. The social and economic factors do influence health care and improvement in social and economical conditions of people cannot only improve the health in community but also promote better use of health resources.
2. Social status in implication of health care as right:
3. A. If people in community are illiterate; they may not understand the need and importance of treating diseases with modern medicine. They may refuse to take treatment or may not be willing to come for follow-up. An educated person may understand and utilize his fundamental rights better.

   B. An educated person will have good job and can access health care facilities provided by government as mostly those working in government set up are insured with Central Government Health Scheme, Employees State Insurance Scheme, AYUSHMAN Bharat Health Scheme, etc. Employed individuals can make better choices about education, child care, food, shelter, health care, etc. Good housing, clean surrounding, consumption of healthy food and seeking medical care during illness are the chain followed by financially well sustained family.

   C. Better social connects are fundamentally helping in people being healthy as they have better mental frame of mind as well as they may get easy information regarding health schemes from their social network.

ECONOMICAL IMPLICATIONS

The financial condition of health care beneficiary as well as those delivering (government/private hospitals) has direct influence on implications of health care utilization as fundamental right.

Key Points

1. The economic condition of people impede them to invest in their health; and vice versa poor economic condition does the reverse.

2. Insurance coverage of beneficiary as well as health care provider shall in providing viable and cost effective health care deliver under consensus of health care as fundamental right especially when beneficiary wish to take medical care in private hospital setup.
3. Government initiatives such as investment in tobacco and alcohol prevention program and levying of excise taxes on cigarettes and alcohol are well appreciative initiative which cannot only generate good finances for better utilization for health care services but also provide clean air policies and lessen lung diseases.
4. Financial implication on Government Budget: Approach of government towards providing adequate health resources for all is itself a challenge in implication of health care as fundamental rights. In India, government has been allocating adequate funds for strengthening the public health.

Conclusion: Economics shapes health policies and effective health care delivery.

MISSING LINKS AND THE IMPLICATIONS FOR DOCTORS

Key Points

The missing links which has larger implication in doctors for discharging their duties towards health care are:

1. Integrated care at all levels: Presently facilities of qualified specialist and super-specialist and diagnostic and therapeutic services are missing from primary, secondary and at times even at tertiary health care center. Improving this missing link will help to cater towards peoples fundamental right for health.
2. There is need for comprehensive health care coupled with state sponsored health insurance for all. Though government provide health care facilities for Below Poverty Line Family free of cost; but many middle class people also find it difficult to spend on health. Increased awareness among public for health insurance can be an effective in accessing health care as a fundamental right by all.
3. Private hospitals and private medical practitioners need promoting health and prevention of illness rather than cashless treatment under umbrella of insurance.
4. Counseling patients for availing health care at primary health center or with general practitioners first rather than rushing for specialist care.
5. The social and economic factors do influence health care and improvement in social and economical conditions of people cannot only improve the health in community but also promote better use of health resources.
6. A robust system in which accountability for failure in delivering standard health care, government incentives, and a system to address public with collective actions in health system needs to be established.

7. A legislatively guaranteed right for health in India; will definitely make fair, just and equitable access to health care a legally binding and ensure accountability.

BIBLIOGRAPHY

1. Fleishacker S. A short history of distributive justice. Cambridge (MA): Harvard University Press; 2005.
2. Giesen D. Health care as a right: some practical implications. Med Law. 1994;13(3-4):285-96. PMID: 7968304.
3. Health and human rights: a resource guide. Open Society Foundations. Open Society Institute. 2013. Archived from the original on 20 January 2012. Retrieved 14 June 2013.
4. Healthcare as a human right ... americanbar.org. Retrieved 2 May 2020.
5. https://tdi.dartmouth.edu/news-events/3-examples-how-economics-affects-health-and-health-care
6. https://www.countyhealthrankings.org/explore-health-rankings/county-health-rankings-model/health-factors/social-economic-factors
7. https://www.legalserviceindia.com/legal/article-6620-right-to-healthcare.html
8. https://www.orfonline.org/expert-speak/declaring-the-right-to-health-a-fundamental-right/
9. https://www.themedicportal.com/application-guide/medical-school-interview/medical-ethics/justice/
10. Human rights and health. https://www.who.int/news-room/fact-sheets/detail/human-rights-and-health
11. Kumar R. Right to health: Challenges and Opportunities. Indian J Community Med. 2015 Oct–Dec;40(4):218–22.
12. Nachiket Mor and Anuska Kalita are with the IKP Trust. https://www.thehindu.com/opinion/lead/Missing-links-in-universal-health-care/article59784065.ece
13. National Health Accounts India. Ministry of Health and Family Welfare, Govt. of India, New Delhi, 2009. [Last accessed on 2015, May 22].
14. Sanjay Nikash. Right to Health and Health Care. https://www.legalserviceindia.com/legal/article-6107-right-to-health-and-health-care.html
15. Varkey B. Principles of Clinical Ethics and their Application to Practice. Med Princ Pract 2021;30:17–28.
16. Yamin, Alicia Ely; Gloppen, Siri Gloppen (2011). Litigating Health Rights, Can Courts Bring More Justice to Health? Harvard University Press. ISBN 9780979639555.

Disclaimer: All information in chapter **(Module 2.3)** Health Care as a Right includes but not limited to; and is for information purpose only. The author declares that the sincere attempt has been made to give standard accurate information in the chapter, but it is not a substitute for any legal or professional advice. The readers should seek advice from legal professional if they are seek consultation and advice for any issue associated with health care as a right.

ASSESSMENT

Write a Short Note on

Barriers to implementation of health care as universal right:

Module

2.4

Working in a Health Care Team

Introduction

Background: The student is to be taught regarding health care systems and their methods of functioning. The students need to "tag along" with health care team members get acquainted to their working pattern and understand their perspectives. This ground experience will be helpful for students to understand the need and scope of working in team in hospital setup.

Learning Objectives

The student after reading the chapter and attending the session should be able to:

1. Demonstrate ability to work in a team of peers and superiors.
2. Demonstrate respect in relationship with patients, fellow team members, superiors and other health care workers.

Discussion

Key Points

1. Need for team work: Doctors in clinics and hospitals work in team and are expected to have a congenial working environment dedicated towards welfare of the patients. A respectful behavior towards colleagues and supporting staff is very much required for a team effort are committed towards providing best health care services and generate higher resilience.
2. Do's and don'ts while working with peers
   A. Greeting them on meeting.
   B. Extend your smile as you start your work.
   C. Always remember that every human has inherent importance and has the right for being treated with dignity.

D. Give autonomy to junior colleagues but instruct to consult before final decision is made regarding the management of patient.
E. Never over-monitor and poke your nose in every taught and action your peers makes.
F. Never undermine your peers capabilities or have distrust in them, never criticize them in back and never insult, disrespect and depress them showing your supremacy of your knowledge and skills. Rather guide and help them in practice.
G. Discuss about patients disease and management and plan your protocol.
H. Listening carefully to suggestions of peers, extend words of encouragement and gratitude, share information and take home the best of knowledge, information and skills while interacting with your peers.
I. Always shared responsibility and be accountable in case of mistakes in a high-quality teamwork.
J. Work together, grow together and becoming team leader should be the goal.

Do's and Don'ts while Working with Subordinates and Supporting Staff in Team Work

A. Greet and introduce oneself to the team members.
B. Explain regarding task to be carried out and explain role and responsibility of each member.
C. Instruct team members with conversation being objective oriented rather than subjective.
D. Discuss to find out if your instructions are well understood.
E. Develop rapport with team members and call them by their names.
F. Have an assertive and commanding tone at time so that team member take work seriously.
G. See your communication is understood and have a planned further communicating procedure for regular feedback.
H. Support your staff in case of mistakes and rectify the wrong.
I. Appreciate your team for good work and support their moral.
J. Be welcoming to staff suggestions and perspective.
K. In conflict situation do not waste time accusing staff for their wrong but carry every task in welfare of patients.

Do's and Don'ts while Working with Superiors

A. Always greet your senior with respect.
B. Be smiling and vocal while you interact with your seniors.
C. Always ensure that dignity of your senior is duly maintained. Never criticize or look down upon your seniors in their absence.

D. The autonomy given by senior to you in working should be acknowledged but do consult them before final decision is made regarding the management of patient.
E. Never poke your nose in every taught and action of your seniors.
F. Never undermine your seniors capabilities or have distrust in them, never criticize them in back and never insult and disrespect them in practice.
G. Discuss about patients disease and management with seniors in case of doubt.
H. Listening carefully to suggestions of seniors, share information and take home the best of knowledge, information and skills while interacting with them.
I. Always shared responsibility and be accountable in case of mistakes in a high-quality teamwork.
J. Work together, grow together, walk in shoes of your ideal seniors and becoming team leader should be the goal.

ASSUMING LEADERSHIP ROLE

1. Treat your peers and subordinates including your paramedic staff with respect.
2. Extend your greeting when you meet them.
3. Set an example for all junior staff by your sincerity, dedication and devotion towards your work.
4. Be punctual and on time at your workplace.
5. Listen carefully to your patients, peers, subordinates and supporting staff.
6. Welcome noble taught and ideas and always remain open to any inputs.
7. Providing autonomy to all junior staff.
8. Encouraging and reminding the team regarding value of the organization or hospital setup you are working.
9. Developing rapport with all junior staff be concerned regarding their personal lives.
10. Supporting peers, subordinates and supporting staff in critical situations.
11. Acknowledge and appreciate your peers, subordinates and supporting staff always.

Do's and Don'ts while Interacting with Patients

1. Develop rapport with your patients. Call by their names. Collect some basic information regarding your patient's job and family.
2. Extend your smile and be considerate towards your patients.
3. Listen to patients complain carefully.
4. Examine patient and spend some time in explaining the patient his health condition and management protocol.
5. Record patient health information and current medical history carefully.
6. Suggest investigations which are necessary and consultations with other specialist if condition of patient warrants so.
7. Maintain confidentiality of patient's health information and record.
8. Have patient written consent for any diagnostic, therapeutic or surgical intervention.
9. Explain the patient regarding follow-up on discharge.
10. Instruct all team members which include junior consultant and nursing staff who have been with you when you have examined the patient regarding management protocol so that patient receives timely intervention during follow-up.

TEAM-BASED HEALTH CARE PRINCIPLES

The principles of a team-based health care include:

1. **Shared goals:** Every team member should be aware of task to be carried out and expected desired outcome.
2. **Clear roles:** The roles and responsibilities of each team member are well defined.
3. **Effective communication:** Chain of effective communication should exist among team members.
4. **Measurable outcomes:** Ensure and record patients recovery for future reference as it can be guiding evidence as well it also denotes the successful working of the team.

Benefits of Teamwork

1. Enhances coordination for effective health care delivery.
2. Appropriate and efficient use of health resources and health care services.
3. Improves communication skills and helps achieving professional excellence.

4. Patients get satisfied, feel encouraged and find solace by efforts made by team members in serving hem.
5. It improves health outcomes and medical errors are reduced.

BIBLIOGRAPHY

1. Babiker A, El Husseini M, Al Nemri A, Al Frayh A, Al Juryyan N, Faki MO, Assiri A, Al Saadi M, Shaikh F, Al Zamil F. Health care professional development: Working as a team to improve patient care. Sudan J Paediatr, 2014;14(2):9–16. PMID: 27493399; PMCID: PMC4949805.
2. http://www.adkhospital.mv/en/page/policies/respect-for-colleagues-guideline
3. Mitchell P, Wynia M, Golden R, McNellis B, Okun S, Webb CE, et al. Core Principles and Values of Effective Team-Based Health Care Discussion Paper. Washington, DC: Institute of Medicine, 2012.
4. World Health Organization. Being an effective team player Available from: URL: http://www.who.int/patientsafety/education/curriculum/who_mc_topic-4.pdf Accessed 2 Decemeber 2014.

ASSIGNMENTS

1. A "tag along" session (4 hours)

The students are instructed to spend time with nurses, technicians and attendant staff, observe their work, their interactions, conduct a small interview with them and write a narrative based on this. (Interview them and collect information regarding their views and opinion about team work and note your findings below.)

Record Interview with Nurses:

____

____

____

____

____

____

____

____

____

____

Interview with Technician:

Interview with Attendant Staff:

Carry a small group discussion in which students will discuss their observations and findings experiences of interviewing staff, and their reflections about what must be done by them to work as an integral part of the health care team. Students to document small group discussion below:

Formative Assessment: Teachers to assess the student participation in session II by evaluating submitted narrative.

Module

2.5

Bioethics Continued: Case Studies on Patient Autonomy and Decision Making

Background: It is important to learn principles of bioethics with case scenario as this will deepen his understanding and the students will be guided by the facilitator to arise at an evidence-based conclusion. The students will learn the details of autonomy and decision making in this module. The case study discussed in the chapter is self designed for giving insight regarding the topic. The teacher can formulate case study from practical experience or live situation in their setup for teaching concepts to the students.

Learning Objectives: The student should be able to:

Identify, discuss and defend medicolegal, sociocultural and ethical issues pertaining to patient autonomy, rights of patients and shared responsibility between doctor and patients in health care.

Discussion

Patient Autonomy, Patient Rights and shared responsibility in health care.

Patient Autonomy

Key Points

1. Autonomy is defined as the quality or state of being self-governing; a self-directing freedom and especially moral independence or a self-governing state. It also means an opportunity which has been given to an individual to live as per his/her own reasoning and motives.
2. As a concept in health patients autonomy refer to their own free will to make decision pertaining to management of his illness, investigation, medication and future course of management and this may not necessarily match with doctors opinion.

3. The doctors must try to explain the potential danger and consequences to patient even if they have refused to take the treatment. The patient is permitted or discharged against medical advice and so mentioned on the case sheet.
4. Attempt made by doctors or patient to pressurize the patient to undertake some treatment is like violation of patient's right to autonomy.

Patient Rights

The commonly practiced patient rights are enlisted below.

1. **Informed consent**
   A. The right to informed consent is a entitlement of patient to be informed regarding of potential harm which may occur to patients own body when he/she is offered medical care. The second part of informed consent foresees that the patient's right to autonomy regarding their treatment is not infringed or violated.
   B. The patients under principle of informed consent must be informed regarding the nature of the diagnostic procedure/ medication/therapy/proposed surgery, etc. the risks and benefits associated with these, the alternatives available treatment modalities and risks and benefits associated with the available alternative modalities.
2. **Confidentiality:** The doctors under medical ethics are bounded to keep the patients illness detail confidential. This principle of confidentiality also grant autonomy to patients as now can control over to decide who can have access to know his/ her health condition. The exceptions to confidentiality which can harm patient or public can be disclosed by doctor to state authorities especially in case of infectious diseases such sexually transmitted infections such as human papillomavirus, gonorrhea, HIV/AIDS, syphilis, etc.
3. **Continuity of health care with doctor:** The patient has right to choose if whether he wishes to continue treatment with particular doctor or seek another. The patient can accept or refuse referrals to specialists and may prefer home treatment.
4. Patient has a right to be treated justly, respectfully and without any discrimination.
5. Patient and their relatives have right to receive information about the medical care which the patient is receiving at any course of time.

6. Patient under his right to autonomy has right to refuse treatment.
7. Patients are to be free from any physical restraints unless there is chance of harm to patient himself or their relatives.
8. Patient has a right to view his medical records and obtain a copy of it at time of discharge.
9. Patient has a right to ask for clarification and explanations about bills.
10. Patients have a right to ask for providing advanced directives against their medical care management.

Shared responsibility between doctor and patients in health care. There is shared responsibility between doctors and patient as they have a common goal of faster health recovery on being provided standard medical care. In this regard it is important that:

1. Patient should be truthful in explaining their health condition and concern if any to the doctor while doctors must welcome patient and address them whenever the patient has doubts, complains or concern.
2. Patient should reveal to doctor complete health history of his present and past, treatment received, hospitalization history, personal history and addiction and family history of illnesses. Doctor must analyze patient in lines of his complete medical history and provide the best standard medical care available.
3. Patient should reveal to doctor under joint responsibility if or not the medication and instructions are followed regularly or not. Doctor may reassess and change treatment strategy in interest of patient welfare.
4. Patients must cooperate with resident doctors and medical students as it aids in learning of trainee doctors but doctors should ensure that there act do not cause discomfort to the patient.
5. Patients must discuss if any financial constraint is there vice versa doctor can arrange few sample medicine if available or alter available best treatment in their hospital set up.
6. Patients should follow lifestyle advices for preventing occurrence of any chronic illness in them.
7. Patient and doctor should not involve in any medical fraud such as spurious clinical trial or organ donation for financial gains.
8. Infectious disease patient should abide by the doctors instruction and avoid causing harm to public.

9. Patients should report any illegal activities conducted by doctor such as sex determination and revealing to patient or multiple termination of pregnancy after 12 weeks (unless clinically justified) to medical licensing authorities.

Paternalism versus Autonomy

Paternalism refers to promotion and restoration of health of patient by providing good medical care and assuming responsibilities for the delivered health care. While autonomy respects patients right to self determine and make decision regarding their health management and so also respecting the patients integrity and decision and eventually it is protecting human rights.

Full Complete Disclosure

This pertains to obligation of doctor to disclose information that any of a reasonable person expects to have for making right decision making. This may lead to patient refusing treatment with doctor, though the doctor believes is in the patient's interest. While the concept of full disclosure as practiced in Western countries states that it is must on part of a doctor to disclose fully the medical errors if occurred by act of omission that which has cause unnecessary harm to patients and doctor is expected to answer the questions of the patients and family members of the patient, and offer financial compensation to the injured party. In lines the compensation in India is decided under Consumer Protection Act.

Moreover, under provision of therapeutic privilege a doctor can withhold complete disclosure if he thinks that the disclosure may affect the patient's emotional and physical condition. But the therapeutic privilege needs to be fully understood in terms of medical law and ethics and needs to be applied as per the law of the country.

BIBLIOGRAPHY

1. Autonomy. https://www.merriam-ebster.com/dictionary/autonomy
2. Chapman CB. Stratton vs. Swanlond: the fourteenth-century ancestor of the law of malpractice. Pharos Alpha Omega Alpha Honor Med Soc. 1982 Fall;45(4):20–4.
3. Emanuel EJ, Emanuel LL. Four models of the physician–patient relationship. JAMA. 1992 Apr 22-29;267(16):2221–6.

4. Hossfeld, George MD Full Disclosure Policies: Risk for Physicians? https://journals.lww.com/em-news/fulltext/2011/04061/full_disclosure_policies__risk_for_physicians_.1.aspx
5. Informed Consent: https://journalofethics.ama-assn.org/article/informed-consent-what-must-physician-disclose-patient/2012–07
6. INTERNATIONAL code of medical ethics (World Medical Associaion, London, October 1949). Madjalah Kedokt Indones. 1959 Oct;9:462.
7. Loh A, Simon D, Wills CE, Kriston L, Niebling W, Härter M. The effects of a shared decision-making intervention in primary care of depression: a cluster-randomized controlled trial. Patient Educ Couns. 2007 Aug;67(3):324–32.
8. Medical Ethics Code. https://code-medical-ethics.ama-assn.org/ethics-opinions/patient-responsibilities
9. Olejarczyk JP, Young M. Patient Rights And Ethics. [Updated 2022 Sep 18]. In: StatPearls [Internet]. Treasure Island (FL): StatPearls Publishing; Jan, 2022. Available from: https://www.ncbi.nlm.nih.gov/books/NBK538279/
10. Pelto-Piri V, Engström, K, Engström I. Paternalism, autonomy and reciprocity: ethical perspectives in encounters with patients in psychiatric in-patient care. BMC Med Ethics 2013;14:49. https://doi.org/10.1186/1472-6939-14-49
11. Physician and Patient; or a Practical View of the Mutual Duties, Relations, and Interests of the Medical Profession and the Community. Br Foreign Med Chir Rev. 1850 Oct;6(12):503–10.
12. Stacey D, Légaré F, Lewis K, Barry MJ, Bennett CL, Eden KB, Holmes-Rovner M, Llewellyn-Thomas H, Lyddiatt A, Thomson R, Trevena L. Decision aids for people facing health treatment or screening decisions. Cochrane Database Syst Rev. 2017 Apr 12;4:CD001431.
13. van Erp WS, Lavrijsen JC, Vos PE, Bor H, Laureys S, Koopmans RT. The vegetative state: prevalence, misdiagnosis, and treatment limitations. J Am Med Dir Assoc. 2015 Jan;16(1):85.e9–85.e14.
14. Wilson CD, Probe RA. Shared Decision-making in Orthopaedic Surgery. J Am Acad Orthop Surg. 2020 Dec. 01;28(23):e1032-e1041.
15. Young M, Wagner A. StatPearls [Internet]. StatPearls Publishing; Treasure Island (FL): May 5, 2022. Medical Ethics. [PubMed]

Disclaimer: All information in chapter **(Module 2.5)** Bioethics Continued: Case Studies on Patient Autonomy and Decision Making includes but not limited to; and is for information purpose only. The author declares that the sincere attempt has been made to give standard accurate information in the chapter, but it is not a substitute for any legal or professional advice. The readers should seek advice from legal professional if they are seek consultation and advice for any issue associated with patient autonomy and decision making.

ASSIGNMENT I: INTRODUCTION AND GROUP FORMATION (1 hour)

The student should be introduced to term paternalism, autonomy and reciprocity, informed consent and full disclosure. Further they may be instructed regarding activities and groups to be formed. The students should note instructions below.

ASSIGNMENT II: CASE INTRODUCTION (1 hour)

Case: The students are instructed to evaluate case below.

Mr Rakesh Kumar, a 55-year-old male presented with complains of increase urge of passing urine, increase frequency of urination and discomfort in emptying bladder and one go. His PSA was increased and on biopsy of prostrate tissue he was diagnosed as case of prostatic carcinoma. He was accompanied by his wife. He is brought to the surgeon who notices that diagnosis is overwritten as benign prostatic hypertrophy after whitening the space. The surgeon guesses a foul play. Wife of patient tells doctor that as my husband will not be able to handle stress I have googled to find suitable replacement to word cancer and done so. I want you to tell my husband that he has benign prostatic hypertrophy. He is waiting in OPD room. I think said surgeon that let's discuss first before we call the husband.

Points for discussion

1. Does the patient have a right to know their diagnosis?
2. What should the patient be told about their diagnosis, therapy and prognosis?
3. How much should be told to a patient about their illness?
4. Are there exceptions to full disclosure?
5. Can family members request withholding of information from patient?

The students can discuss the case under guidance of mentor and write there discussion points.

ASSIGNMENT III: SELF-DIRECTED LEARNING (2 hours)

The students can read various research papers and surf through genuine approved website and record finding below:

Papers may be referred to:

1. Olejarczyk JP, Young M. Patient Rights And Ethics. [Updated 2022 Sep 18]. In: StatPearls [Internet]. Treasure Island (FL): StatPearls Publishing; 2022 Jan. Available from: https://www.ncbi.nlm.nih.gov/books/NBK538279/
2. Young M, Wagner A. StatPearls [Internet]. StatPearls Publishing; Treasure Island (FL): May 5, 2022. Medical Ethics [PubMed].
3. Chapman CB. Stratton vs Swanlond: the fourteenth-century ancestor of the law of malpractice. Pharos Alpha Omega Alpha Honor Med Soc. 1982 Fall;45(4):20–4.

4. Emanuel EJ, Emanuel LL. Four models of the physician-patient relationship. JAMA. 1992 Apr 22–29;267(16):2221–6.
5. Informed Consent: https://journalofethics.ama-assn.org/article/informed-consent-what-must-physician-disclose-patient/2012–07
6. Hossfeld, George MD. Full Disclosure Policies: Risk for Physicians? https://journals.lww.com/em-news/fulltext/2011/04061/full_disclosure_policies__risk_for_physicians_.1.aspx
7. Pelto-Piri V, Engström K, Engström I. Paternalism, autonomy and reciprocity: ethical perspectives in encounters with patients in psychiatric in-patient care. BMC Med Ethics 2013;14:49. https://doi.org/10.1186/1472-6939-14-49
8. Medical Ethics Code. https://code-medical-ethics.ama-assn.org/ethics-opinions/patient-responsibilities
9. Autonomy. https://www.merriam-ebster.com/dictionary/autonomy

Points for discussion:

1. Does the patient have a right to know the diagnosis?
   Yes, the patient has a right to know the diagnosis as per the principle of informed consent as specified under the recommended NMC Code of Ethics. Rakesh must know regarding his state of prostatic carcinoma.
2. What should the patient be told about the diagnosis, therapy and prognosis?
   Yes, the patient must be told about the diagnosis, therapy and prognosis expect under therapeutic previleges.
3. How much should be told to a patient about their illness?
   Complete and full disclosure about his condition must be told to patient.
4. Are there exceptions to full disclosure?
   Yes, moreover under provision of therapeutic privilege a doctor can withhold complete disclosure if he thinks that the disclosure may affect the patient's emotional and physical condition.
5. Can family members request withholding of information from patient?

No family members cannot request a doctor from withholding any information from patient as is contradictory under law but as under provision of therapeutic privilege a doctor can withhold complete disclosure if he thinks that the disclosure may affect the patient's emotional and physical condition. But forging document by changing diagnosis though done by patients relative in this case is an offence.

The students can discuss case as detailed in IMG competency syllabus as detailed in beginning of chapter.

ASSESSMENT

1. **Formative:** The students are to be assessed based on their active participation in the above sessions.

2. **Summative:** Students are instructed to write short notes on:

1. Define patient autonomy.

2. Contrast autonomy and paternalism.

3. **What are the responsibilities of patients and doctors in shared decision making?**

4. What is full and reasonable disclosure?

Module

2.6

Bioethics: Case Studies on Autonomy and Decision Making

Background: This module shall introduce the student to various other issues in autonomy including competence and capacity to make decisions. The case study discussed in the chapter is self-designed for giving insight regarding the topic. The teacher can formulate case study from practical experience or live situation in their setup for teaching concepts to the students.

Learning Objectives: The student should be able to:
Identify, discuss and defend medicolegal, sociocultural and ethical issues pertaining to refusal of care including do not resuscitate and withdrawal of life support.

Medicolegal, sociocultural and ethical issues pertaining to refusal of care including do not resuscitate and withdrawal of life support: Shared Decision Making.

Key Points

Global Concept

1. There is moral and legal obligation and responsibility of a qualified medical practitioner to have a complete and full disclosure of patient's health condition, prognosis and in case of deteriorating prognosis of the patient and if required with the patient's relative, especially when further medical management and support appears not useful to save patient's life. The benefits and burdens of available therapeutic options and the justified action to allow natural death must be discussed by the doctor (qualified medical practitioner).
2. The doctor (qualified medical practitioner) must inform patient/family members and obtain consent about management strategies of comfort

care and limitation of life-prolonging interventions as condition of patient is critical.

3. The doctor (qualified medical practitioner) shall make a shared decision along with patient/relatives in such a grim prognosis and patients choices be duly respected considering the autonomy right of the patient.
4. All conversation and counseling of patient / relatives should be documented and recorded by the doctor (qualified medical practitioner).
5. The doctor (qualified medical practitioner) shall continue life support till the death of the patient.
6. Euthanasia: It encompasses the practice of intentionally ending life to eliminate pain and suffering. The concept of active euthanasia or physician assisted end to life is not yet legalized in India.
7. The Supreme Court of India in its landmark judgment legalized passive euthanasia on ninth of March 2018 by withdrawal of life support in patient in permanent vegetative state of life. This landmark judgment was given by Supreme Court of India in a plea of Pinki Virani's plea case which was filed in December 2009 under the Constitutional provisions of "Next Friend" for her friend nurse Aruna Ramchandra Shanbaug who was a nurse in the KEM Hospital, Mumbai and was assaulted and later strangulated by ward boy, Sohanlal Bhartha Valmiki in November 1973 due to which she lived in vegetative state for 42 years and died in 2015. The Supreme Court of India specified two such irreversible conditions to permit Passive Euthanasia in its 2011 Law and this included brain-dead patient for whom the ventilator can be switched or taken and those in a Persistent Vegetative State (PVS).
8. In decision making capacity represents a person's inherent ability to make informed decisions and as to providing informed consent regarding his / her welfare. Competency is a universal assessment and a legal determination of facts which is made by a judge in court.
9. To conclude the three essential elements in decision making are recognizing, identifying and acknowledging that there is need to make decision; know and understand the best available evidence; and incorporate patient's values and preferences in the process of decision making.

BIBLIOGRAPHY

1. Andy Odden, Joyeeta G. Dastidar. How Do I Determine if My Patient has Decision-Making Capacity? https://www.the-hospitalist.org/hospitalist/article/124731/how-do-i-determine-if-my-patient-has-decision-making-capacity
2. Buckley TA, Joynt GM, Tan PY, Cheng CA, Yap FH. Limitation of life support: Frequency and practice in a Hong Kong intensive care unit. Crit Care Med 2004;32:415–20.
3. Burns J, Edwards J, Johnson J, Cassem NH, Troug RD. Do-not-resuscitate order after 25 years. Crit Care Med. 2003;31:1543–50.

4. Eliasson AH, Parker JM, Shorr AF, Babb KA, Harris R, Aaronson BA, et al. Impediments to writing do-not-resuscitate orders. Arch Intern Med 1999;159:2213–8.
5. Gaikwad A, Acharya S. The Future of Palliative Treatment in India: A Review. Cureus 2022 Sep 23;14(9):e29502.
6. Ganzini L, Volicer L, Nelson WA, Fox E, Derse AR. Ten myths about decisionmaking capacity. J Am Med Dir Assoc 2004;5(4):263–7.
7. Hayes S, Stewart K. The role of audit in making do not resuscitate decisions. J Eval Clin Pract 1998;5:305–12.
8. Kamat V. Guiding light at the end of the tunnel. Indian J Med Ethics 2006;3:103–4.
9. Kaveri Mayra, Zoë Matthews, Jane Sandall (2021) 'Surrogate decision making' in India for women competent to consent and choose during childbirth, Agenda, 35:3, 92–103, DOI: 10.1080/10130950.2021.1958549
10. Légaré F, Witteman HO. Shared decision making: examining key elements and barriers to adoption into routine clinical practice. Health Aff (Millwood). 2013 Feb;32(2):276-84. doi: 10.1377/hlthaff.2012.1078. PMID: 23381520.
11. Mani RK, Amin P, Chawla R, Divatia JV, Kapadia F, Khilnani P, Myatra SN, Prayag S, Rajagopalan R, Todi SK, Uttam R. Guidelines for end-of-life and palliative care in Indian intensive care units' ISCCM consensus Ethical Position Statement. Indian J Crit Care Med 2012 Jul;16(3):166–81.
12. Mani RK, Amin P, Chawla R, Divatia JV, Kapadia F, Khilnani P, et al. ISCCM position statement: Limiting life-prolonging interventions and providing palliative care towards the end of life in Indian intensive care units. Indian J Crit Care Med 2005;9:96–107.
13. Rao MJ. Legal issues related to the limitation of life support: A review of the international legal process. Indian J Crit Care Med 2005;9:115–9.
14. Salins NS, Pai SG, Vidyasagar M, Sobhana M. Ethics and medico-legal aspects of "not for resuscitation". Indian J Palliat Care 2010 May;16(2):66–9.
15. Sharma H, Jagdish V, Anusha P, Bharti S. End-of-life care: Indian perspective. Indian J Psychiatry 2013 Jan;55(Suppl 2):S293–8.
16. Tomlinson T, Brody H. Ethics and communications in do-not-resuscitate orders. N Engl J Med 1986;318:43–6.

Disclaimer: All information in chapter **(Module 2.6)** Bioethics: Case Studies on Autonomy and Decision Making includes but not limited to; and is for information purpose only. The author declares that the sincere attempt has been made to give standard accurate information in the chapter, but it is not a substitute for any legal or professional advice. The reader should seek advice from legal professional if they are seek consultation and advice for any issue associated with patient autonomy and decision making.

ASSIGNMENT I: CASE INTRODUCTION (1 hour)

Teacher must introduce the case and guide them for basic principle in medical practice.

Case

Patient Rekha who is 84 year is suffering from gallstone disease. Her husband died two years ago due to acute renal failure. He was resuscitated for nearly 30 minutes by doctor and Rekha was disgusted, pained and scared by thumping which she felt was cruel. He eventually died. Rekha recently developed Alzheimer's disease. She is conscious and vocal at times but forgets regarding where she has kept her things or sometimes even ask her servant for breakfast twice. Later she got admitted for cholecystitis with complain of nausea and vomiting and pain in upper right quadrant of abdomen. She has also seen her sister dying do to burns in past and is nervous as she remembers the terminal aid feeding by Ryles tube and all intra-venous therapy; and she is anxious what she has to go through. She explains to her doctor not any chest resuscitation or tube feeding for her. The abdominal ultrasound has confirmed gallstone and doctor explains regarding required surgical intervention. Her son has accompanied her for admission and wants to know patients prognosis from doctor. In this case address the question below as per Code of Medical Ethics.

Points for discussion

1. Extent of patient autonomy.
2. Elements in decision making: Competency vs capacity.
3. Surrogacy in decision making.
4. Autonomy vs beneficence.
5. How much does family wishes count?
6. Legal, ethical and social aspects of 'do-not-resuscitate'.

ASSIGNMENT II: SELF-DIRECTED LEARNING (2 hours)

The students may go through following reference paper and self study

1. Mani RK, Amin P, Chawla R, Divatia JV, Kapadia F, Khilnani P, et al. ISCCM position statement: Limiting life-prolonging interventions and providing palliative care towards the end of life in Indian intensive care units. Indian J Crit Care Med. 2005;9: 96–107.

2. Burns J, Edwards J, Johnson J, Cassem NH, Troug RD. Do-not-resuscitate order after 25 years. Crit Care Med 2003;31:1543–50.
3. Buckley TA, Joynt GM, Tan PY, Cheng CA, Yap FH. Limitation of life support: Frequency and practice in a Hong Kong intensive care unit. Crit Care Med 2004;32:415–20.
4. Salins NS, Pai SG, Vidyasagar M, Sobhana M. Ethics and medico-legal aspects of "not for resuscitation". Indian J Palliat Care 2010 May 16(2):66–9.
5. Mani RK, Amin P, Chawla R, Divatia JV, Kapadia F, Khilnani P, Myatra SN, Prayag S, Rajagopalan R, Todi SK, Uttam R. Guidelines for end-of-life and palliative care in Indian intensive care units' ISCCM consensus Ethical Position Statement. Indian J Crit Care Med 2012 Jul;16(3):166–81.
6. Ganzini L, Volicer L, Nelson WA, Fox E, Derse AR. Ten myths about decision-making capacity. J Am Med Dir Assoc 2004;5(4): 263–7.
7. Légaré F, Witteman HO. Shared decision making: examining key elements and barriers to adoption into routine clinical practice. Health Aff (Millwood). 2013 Feb;32(2):276-84. doi: 10.1377/hlthaff.2012.1078. PMID: 23381520.
8. Andy Odden, Joyeeta G Dastidar. How do I determine if my patient has decision-making capacity? https://www.the-hospitalist.org/hospitalist/article/124731/how-do-i-determine-if-my-patient-has-decision-making-capacity

Write the unique observations below:

___

___

___

___

___

___

___

___

___

___

___

ASSIGNMENT III: ANCHORING LECTURE (1 hour)

As detailed in discussion: Students may take teachers notes below:

ASSIGNMENT IV: DISCUSSION AND CLOSURE OF CASE (1 hour)

Points for discussion

1. **Extent of patient autonomy**

   Patient has right to autonomy to accept or reject any treatment modalities.

   [Patient has explained to her doctor that not to perform any chest resuscitation or tube feeding for her; so doctor needs to re-discuss and resolve her queries and need to abide by patients autonomy rights with exception under emergency]

2. **Elements in decision making: Competency vs capacity.**

   In decision making: Capacity represents a person's inherent ability to make informed decisions and as to providing informed consent regarding his/her welfare. (Patient Rekha had capacity to make decision regarding her health and treatment modality.) Competency is a universal assessment and a legal determination of facts which is made by a judge in court.

3. **Surrogacy in decision making**

   The 'surrogate decision maker' is a guardian who is entrusted to make appropriate decision regarding patient health and management modalities as patients are not in condition to make suitable decision due to their mental illness or are in incapacitated condition.

4. **Autonomy vs beneficence**

   Autonomy is patient's right to except treatment and consent for same while beneficence is an act of charity, mercy, and kindness of doctor (qualified medical practitioner) and his moral obligation to ensure and safeguard the health of the people. [Rekha's right versus surgeon dutiful act of offering standard medical care.]

5. **How much does family wishes count?**

   Patient's wishes are most important and needed to be adhered to unless the patient is in incapacitated condition, patient is having mental illness or in case of life-threatening emergency conditions when there is no sufficient time to obtain consent the family wishes are to be considered. [In present case Rekha is in capacity to consent.]

6. **Legal, ethical and social aspects of 'Do-not-resuscitate'**

   Euthanasia: It encompasses the practice of intentionally ending life to eliminate pain and suffering. The concept of active euthanasia or physician assisted end to life is not yet legalized in India. The Supreme Court of India in its landmark judgment legalized passive euthanasia on ninth of March 2018 by withdrawal of life support in patient in permanent vegetative state of life. This landmark judgment was given by Supreme Court of India in a plea of Pinki Virani's case which was filed in December 2009 under the Constitutional provisions of "Next Friend" for her friend nurse Aruna Ramchandra Shanbaug who was a nurse in the KEM Hospital Mumbai and was assaulted and later strangulated by ward boy, Sohanlal Bhartha Valmiki in November 1973 due to which she lived in vegetative state for 42 years and died in 2015. The Supreme Court of India specified two such irreversible conditions to permit Passive Euthanasia in its 2011 Law and this included brain-dead patient for whom the ventilator can be switched or taken off and those in a persistent vegetative state (PVS).

This issue on ethical and social basis has not been found appropriate by various health society and organization.

Additional Assignment: Discuss the Case of IMG Curriculum

ASSESSMENT

1. **Formative:** The student may be assessed based on their active participation in the sessions.
2. **Summative:** Write short notes on:

   a. What determines decision-making capacity and competency.

b. Who has the right to make decisions for a patient who cannot determine for himself?

Module

2.7

Bioethics: Case Studies on Autonomy and Decision Making

Background: This module discusses other issues in autonomy including informed consent and refusal. The case study discussed in the chapter is self designed for giving insight regarding the topic. The teacher can formulate case study from practical experience or live situation in their setup for teaching concepts to the student.

Learning Objectives: The student should be able to:
Identify, describe, discuss and offer a defense in reference to consent and associated medicolegal, sociocultural and ethical issues.

Key Points

1. As per the provision of Article 21 the patient under their right to autonomy can accept or refuse treatment and if willing gives a written consent for accepting any treatment modality.
2. Doctors need to make complete disclosure about patient's disease. Prior to obtaining consent the patient should be told regarding the disease condition, planned treatment, prognosis, risk and benefits of the planned modality of treatment and alternative treatment modalities and risk and benefit about the alternative modality.
3. Informed consent and informed refusal. The doctor needs to obtain consent from patient regarding the treatment after discussing complete treatment protocol, probable risk and benefits and alternative treatment modalities. The disclosure to the patient should be complete regarding the prognosis. Patient has right to refuse treatment. The doctor (qualified medical practitioner) should further initiate discussion to answer queries and resolve patients doubt. If he still refuses the doctor is not under legal binding. All conversations are to be recorded.

4. Autonomy and beneficence concept in consent: Autonomy is patient's right to except treatment and consent for same while beneficence is an act of charity, mercy, and kindness of doctor (qualified medical practitioner) and his moral obligation to ensure and safeguard the health of the people.
5. The informed consent must be informed and voluntary (freely given and not under pressure) and person must be capable to give consent. The patient should be told regarding the disease condition, planned treatment, prognosis, risk and benefits of the planned modality of treatment and alternative treatment modalities and risk and benefit about the alternative modality.
6. Even in clinical research a written consent is to be obtained from participant after informing them regarding basis and objective of research, feasible benefits and risk if any, any possibility of hazards, compensation in case of harm, confidentiality regarding participants identity and preservation of data.
7. Consent is the legal and ethical expression of the basic right of individual to have autonomy and self-determination regarding his/her health.
8. Implied consent refers to consideration that permission has been given to do something and this is inferred from a person's actions (facial expression and verbal cues) rather than explicitly expressed.
9. Various exceptions which are taken into consideration when informed consent is not obtained from patients; but then it has to be taken from spouse/ Kins, etc. (1) the incapacitated condition of the patient, (2) life-threatening emergency conditions when there is no sufficient time to obtain consent.
10. The National Medical Code Ethics formally the Medical Council of India (MCI) directive states that a consent is to be obtained in writing prior to performing an operation.

    The MCI guidelines are pertaining to operations and not treatments. In case of treatments, the guidelines to be followed are:
    a. In routine treatment the implied consent is sufficient
    b. In detailed treatment, oral consent is required
    c. In complex treatment modalities written express consent is to be obtained.
11. Any individual above 18 years of age, having sound mind, and have not been disqualified under any law can give consent as per Indian Majority Act.
12. As per directive of Supreme Court of India if consent is for diagnostic procedure then it is for diagnostic procedure only and not for surgical or any other intervention.
13. The obligation of a doctor to offer standard medical care to his/her patient is total, absolute, and paramount the apex court opined that a medical practitioner has a duty to offer best standard treat a patient in an emergency condition of patient. This is irrespective of following any formalities, including consent.

BIBLIOGRAPHY

1. Declaration of Helsinki. 1964.
2. Informed Consent: https://www.msdmanuals.com/en-in/home/fundamentals/legal-and-ethical-issues/informed-consent
3. Nandimath OV. Consent and medical treatment: The legal paradigm in India. Indian J Urol. 2009 Jul;25(3):343–7. doi: 10.4103/0970-1591.56202. PMID: 19881130; PMCID: PMC2779959.
4. Regulation 7.16, of Medical Council of India (Professional Conduct, Etiquette and Ethics) Regulations, 2002 (NMC Code of Ethics).
5. Shah P, Thornton I, Turrin D, Hipskind JE. Informed Consent. 2022 Jun 11. In: StatPearls [Internet]. Treasure Island (FL): StatPearls Publishing; 2022 Jan. PMID: 28613577.

Discussion

All information in chapter (Module 2.7 Bioethics continued – Case studies on patient autonomy and decision making) includes but not limited to; and is for information purpose only. The author declares that the sincere attempt has been made to give standard accurate information in the chapter, but it is not a substitute for any legal or professional advice. The reader should seek advice from legal professional if they are seek consultation and advice for any issue associated with patient autonomy and decision making.

ASSIGNMENT I: CASE INTRODUCTION (1 hour)

The teacher to introduce the case and make preliminary discussion

A 48-year-old male patient was admitted to hospital with complaints of acute pain in inguinal region and was diagnosed as obstructive hernia. Surgeon instructed the patient that he has to be immediately operated upon. The patient's father had expired two years back while being operated for acute lower bowel perforation. His mother passed six months back while angioplasty was been conducted. The patient has phobia for operation and ask doctor do any other treatment or apply special abdominal belt (corset). The doctor gets wild and instructs patient that no more your nonsense, I am best surgeon of the town, instruct nurse to shift patient to operation theater. Patient further wished to know regarding management protocol. Doctor hushes the patient and asks him I am Doctor or you are? If not interested you may go to other hospital.

ASSIGNMENT II: SELF DIRECTED LEARNING (2 hours)

Students to refer the references below

1. 1964. Declaration of Helsinki.
2. Regulation 7.16, Medical Council of India (Professional Conduct, Etiquette and Ethics) Regulations, 2002 (NMC Code of Ethics).
3. Nandimath OV. Consent and medical treatment: The legal paradigm in India. Indian J Urol. 2009 Jul;25(3):343–7. doi: 10.4103/0970-1591.56202. PMID: 19881130; PMCID: PMC2779959.
4. Informed Consent: https://www.msdmanuals.com/en-in/home/fundamentals/legal-and-ethical-issues/informed-consent
5. Shah P, Thornton I, Turrin D, Hipskind JE. Informed Consent. 2022 Jun 11. In: StatPearls [Internet]. Treasure Island (FL): StatPearls Publishing; 2022 Jan. PMID: 28613577.

ASSIGNMENT III: ANCHORING LECTURE (1 hour)

This is based on key points as elaborated in beginning of the chapter

ASSIGNMENT IV: DISCUSSION AND CLOSURE OF CASE (1 hour)

Points for discussion:

1. **Extent of patient autonomy**
   Patient under his right of autonomy can refuse treatment though if he knows that by doing so he may die. But doctors need to re-communicate and assure regarding patients queries and apprehension in best interest of patients health as this patient was having obstructive hernia which is surgical emergency.
2. **Informed consent and informed refusal**
   The doctor (qualified medical practitioner) needs to obtain consent from patient regarding the treatment after discussing complete treatment protocol, probable risk and benefits and alternative treatment modalities. The disclosure to the patient should be complete regarding the prognosis. Patient has right to refuse treatment. The doctor (qualified medical practitioner) should further initiate discussion to answer queries and resolve patients doubt. If he still refuses the doctor is not under legal binding. All conversations are to be recorded. In case of emergency medical condition there is provision of exception of consent in case of incapacitated condition of patient or if the condition which the patient is suffering is life-threatening. Usually consent in such a state is obtained from near relatives.
3. **Conflict between autonomy and beneficence**
   Autonomy is patient's right to except treatment and consent for same while beneficence is an act of charity, mercy, and kindness of doctor (qualified medical practitioner) and his moral obligation to ensure and safeguard the health of the people. [The apprehension of patient and past experience has prompt patient to think about refusing of treatment but surgeons act of beneficence prompts him to operate immediately.]
4. **What should the patient be told about a procedure?**
   The patient should be told regarding the nature of procedure, i.e. reducing strangulated hernia and later surgical repair of hernia, risk and benefits of the planned procedure and alternative treatment modalities if any and risk and benefit about the alternative modality. In present condition surgery is the line of treatment.

5. What must the informed consent include?

It must be informed and voluntary (freely given and not under pressure) and person must be capable to give consent. The patient should be told regarding the disease condition, planned treatment, prognosis, risk and benefits of the planned modality of treatment and alternative treatment modalities and risk and benefit about the alternative modality.

Additional Case: The students can discuss and write the findings of case given in IMG curriculum

ASSESSMENT

1. **Formative:** The student may be assessed based on their active participation in the sessions.

Assessment Report by Teacher

2. **Summative:** Write short questions on:

1. What is informed consent?

2. What is informed refusal?

Module

2.8

What Does it Mean to be Family Member of a Sick Patient?

Background: Doctors interact with patients addressing their human suffering. It is necessary for the grooming upcoming doctors to needs to understand the balanced approach required in patient care, the intricacy of working of support systems of patients, patients expectation and priorities, patients coping stamina and emotions of family members.

Learning Objectives: The student should be able to:

- Demonstrate empathy in patient encounters.
- Patients, their priorities, coping abilities and emotions of families.

Key Points

1. Patients experience anxiety, worry and curiosity when ill and wish to get well faster. The doctors in busy schedule have to address the emotions and feelings of the family members apart from their duties to impart standard medical care to the patients.
2. Patient's priority is to receive consultation and treatment from qualified and empathetic doctors. They expect to be informed by doctor regarding their illness, course of treatment and prognosis. The patients expect the supporting staff such as resident doctor, nurses and attendants to be available at their bed side whenever they have any discomfort. The patients also expect love and affection from his near and dear one. The patients also expect that doctors should give sufficient time towards listening to their complaints and examining them during every visit including follow-up.
3. The patient's coping capability depends on his mental framework, his physical health, his nature of illness and his psychology in which he has been brought up from childhood whenever sick.
4. The three core emotional components usually expressed by chronically ill patient's include fear, sadness and anger. His fear and anger may delay his healing as positive outlook always facilitate positive health outcome.

5. Emotion of family members: The family members of patients are worried and anxious about health of their family member. Research studies have pointed out that two-thirds of family members of patients admitted to intensive care unit had symptoms of depression, anxiety, or post-traumatic stress.
6. Coping strategies of family members:
   a. Problem-solving: The family members seek doctor's advice so that patient's health problem is resolved.
   b. Information seeking: The family members wish to be aware of patient's health, his course of management and his prognosis.
   c. Self-reliance: The family members always that good is in stored and their patient will be cured and healed. An empathic approach of doctors and nurses towards their patient generate a feeling of self reliance and expected positive outcome in their patient's health.
   d. Social and religious support: The family members seek social and religious support to solace for faster recovery of their near one.
   e. Stress and worry: The family members may have stress and may be worried regarding financial implication of illness in case they are poor or middle class family.
   f. Getting accommodated: The family members get accommodated over period of time regarding health issues and outcome of their patients in cases of their patients are chronically ill.
   g. Counselors at hospital setup may help the family members by reducing psychological distress among them.

EMPATHY IN MEDICINE

Key Points

1. Empathy is the ability to understand and share the feelings of another. Doctors when interacting with their patients come to know about the state of mind of their patients, whether they are happy, satisfied, contended or irritated, sad and depressed. Doctors must express their empathy while further managing the patient's illness.
2. The doctors as good communicators must expressed their perception about patient's emotions to them as patients get solace that doctor is empathetic towards their misery and health issue.
3. Doctors who are good listeners do exhibit empathy towards patient.
4. Doctors must show empathy but must not get too much attached emotionally.
5. The budding doctors can be taught how to develop empathy? And this can be achieved by making them react with patients and then have self-reflective writing regarding the incidence. This will gradually generate empathetic emotional responses in them.
6. Doctor's empathetic ability and effective applicability generate excellent therapeutic results.

7. The good empathetic relationship between doctors and patients will help designing a good therapeutic plan as well as it ensures that patient will abide by the treatment.
8. A well understood relation based on empathy between doctors and patient makes them feel secure and trusts on their doctor increases. It also lessens stress and burnout in doctors at workplace and improves quality of life of doctors.
9. It is recommended to use non-verbal cues such as appropriate body movements, tone of voice, and facial expressions by doctors as this reaffirms their empathy.
10. The factors influencing empathy are age of doctor, his mental framework, workload, his family circumstances, his ideologies and beliefs, etc.
11. Reorientation to medical education are periodically needed for the reinforcement of empathetic skill.

BIBLIOGRAPHY

1. Adler HM. The history of the present illness as treatment: who's listening, and why does it matter? J Am Board Fam Pract 1997;10(1): 28–35.
2. Buie DH. Empathy: its nature and limitations. J Am Psychoanal Assocn 1981;29(2):281–307.
3. Harlan EA, Miller J, Costa DK, Fagerlin A, Iwashyna TJ, Chen EP, Lipman K, Valley TS. Emotional Experiences and Coping Strategies of Family Members of Critically Ill Patients. Chest 2020 Oct;158(4): 1464–72.
4. https://journalofethics.ama-assn.org/article/role-empathy-medicine medical-students-perspective/2007–06
5. Jollife D, Farrigthon DP. Development and validation of the basic empathy scale. J Adolesc 2005;29:589–611. doi: 10.1016/j.adolescence. 2005.08.010.
6. Kahrima I, Nural N, Arsal U, Torbas M, Can G, Kasim S. The effect of empathy training on the empathic skills of nurses. Iran Red Crescent Med J 2016;18:1–10.
7. Larson EB, Yao X. Clinical empathy as emotional labor in the patient–physician relationship. JAMA 2005;293(9):1100–6.
8. Oxford English Dictionary Online. Oxford University Press. [(accessed on 15 September 2019)]; Available online: http://oxforddictionaries. com/definition/English/empathyq=empathy
9. Platt FW, Keller VF. Empathic communication: a teachable and learnable skill. J Gen Intern Med 1994;9(4):222–6.
10. Suchman AL, Markakis K, Beckman HB, Frankel R. A model of empathic communication in the medical interview. JAMA 1997;277(8):678–82.

`11. Taigman M. Can empathy and compassion be taught? JEMS 1996; 21(6):42–43, 45–46, 48.

ASSIGNMENTS

Total hours: 6 (includes 2 hours of SDL)

ASSIGNMENT I: HOSPITAL VISIT AND INTERVIEWS (2 hours)

Assign students, a patient admitted in the hospital, and instruct them to interview their family about their patient illnesses, their experience in hospital, and so also reactions, emotions, outlook and expectations they have from hospital authorities such as doctors and nurses. Record your interview of at least two relatives of two different patients:

Patient 1

Patient 2

ASSIGNMENT II

The teacher may arrange a large group discussions with patients' relatives in lecture hall by inviting at least 4 patients. The students to note the discussion (1 hour)

Patient 1

Patient 2

Patient 3

Patient 4

ASSIGNMENT III: SELF-DIRECTED LEARNING (2 hours)

The students shall write a report from reflection based on sessions 1 and 2 and may be shared research papers and articles relevant to topic for self learning.

Reference paper for self-learning

1. Harlan EA, Miller J, Costa DK, Fagerlin A, Iwashyna TJ, Chen EP, Lipman K, Valley TS. Emotional Experiences and Coping Strategies of Family Members of Critically Ill Patients. Chest 2020 Oct;158(4): 1464–72.
2. Larson EB, Yao X. Clinical empathy as emotional labor in the patient-physician relationship. JAMA 2005;293(9):1100–6.
3. https://journalofethics.ama-assn.org/article/role-empathy-medicine-medical-students-perspective/2007–06.
4. Kahrima I, Nural N, Arsal U, Torbas M, Can G, Kasim S. The effect of empathy training on the empathic skills of nurses. Iran Red Crescent Med J 2016;18:1–10.
5. Jollife D, Farrigthon DP. Development and validation of the basic empathy scale. J Adolesc 2005;29:589–611.

Students Report

ASSIGNMENT IV: DISCUSSION AND CLOSURE (1 hour)

The teacher to discuss the topic and assignments and give the student a take home message.

Take Home Message

ASSESSMENT

1. **Formative**

   Grade the student's performance as Excellent/Very Good/Good/Satisfactory/Poor based on their active participation in the sessions and submission of the written narrative.

2. **Summative:** The students are instructed to write short notes on:

   1. **The role of doctors in the community and expectations of society from doctors.**

2. What is empathy? What is the role of empathy in the care of patients?

READER'S NOTES

READER'S NOTES

READER'S NOTES

READER'S NOTES

READER'S NOTES

READER'S NOTES